Dedicated to our ABCs,
especially our Cai Lionheart

Foreword

Dear Reader,

It was a hard, scary day when we got the news our baby had a heart defect. It was the start of a long, painful journey. But we look back on that day and see that we had hope from the beginning.

If you or a loved one is facing something similar, we pray this book will give you a peek into what may lie ahead. Your journey is your own. Your path will be different. You may have a Heart Warrior or a Heart Angel. But there is a beautiful plan of purpose, hope, and love that is unfolding before you.

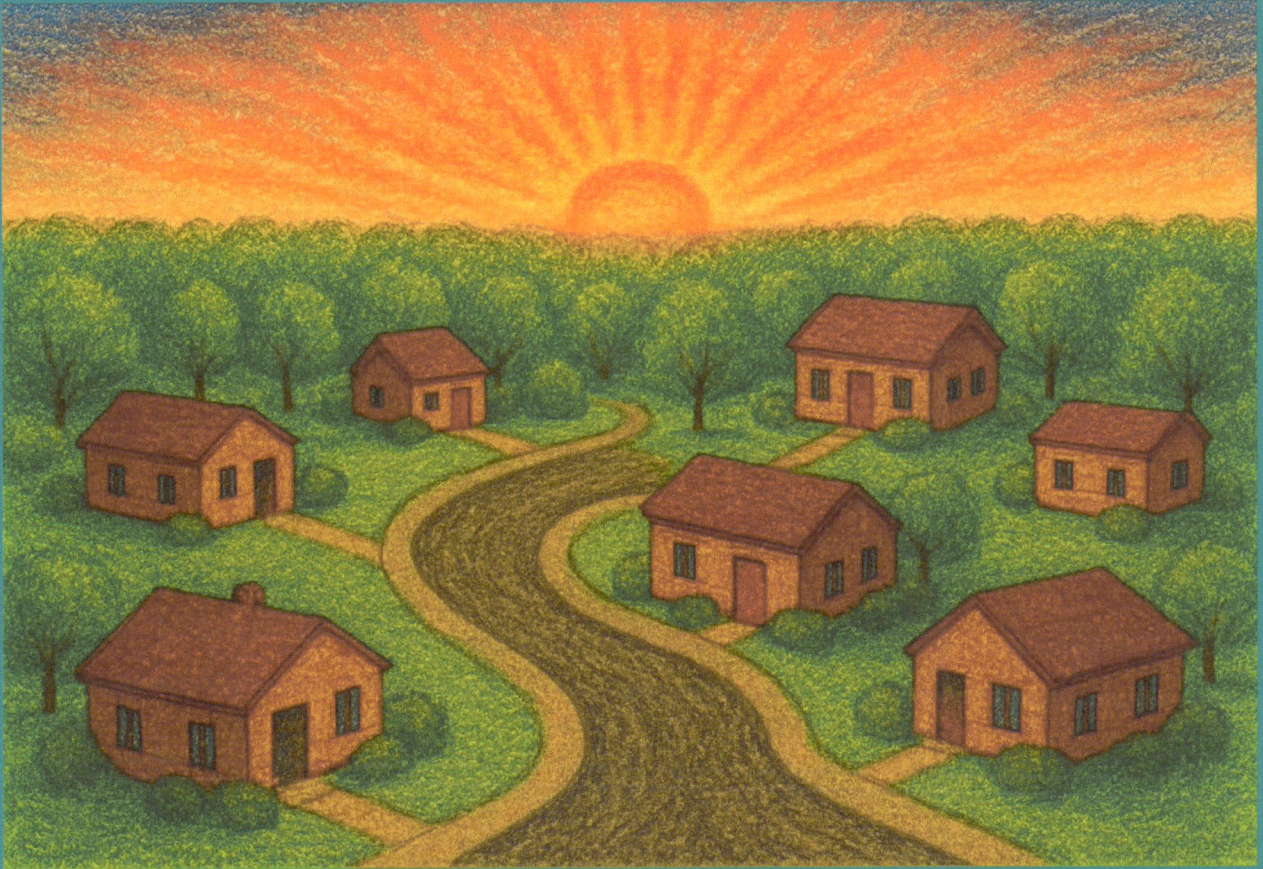

Everything felt steady, we had a normal life.

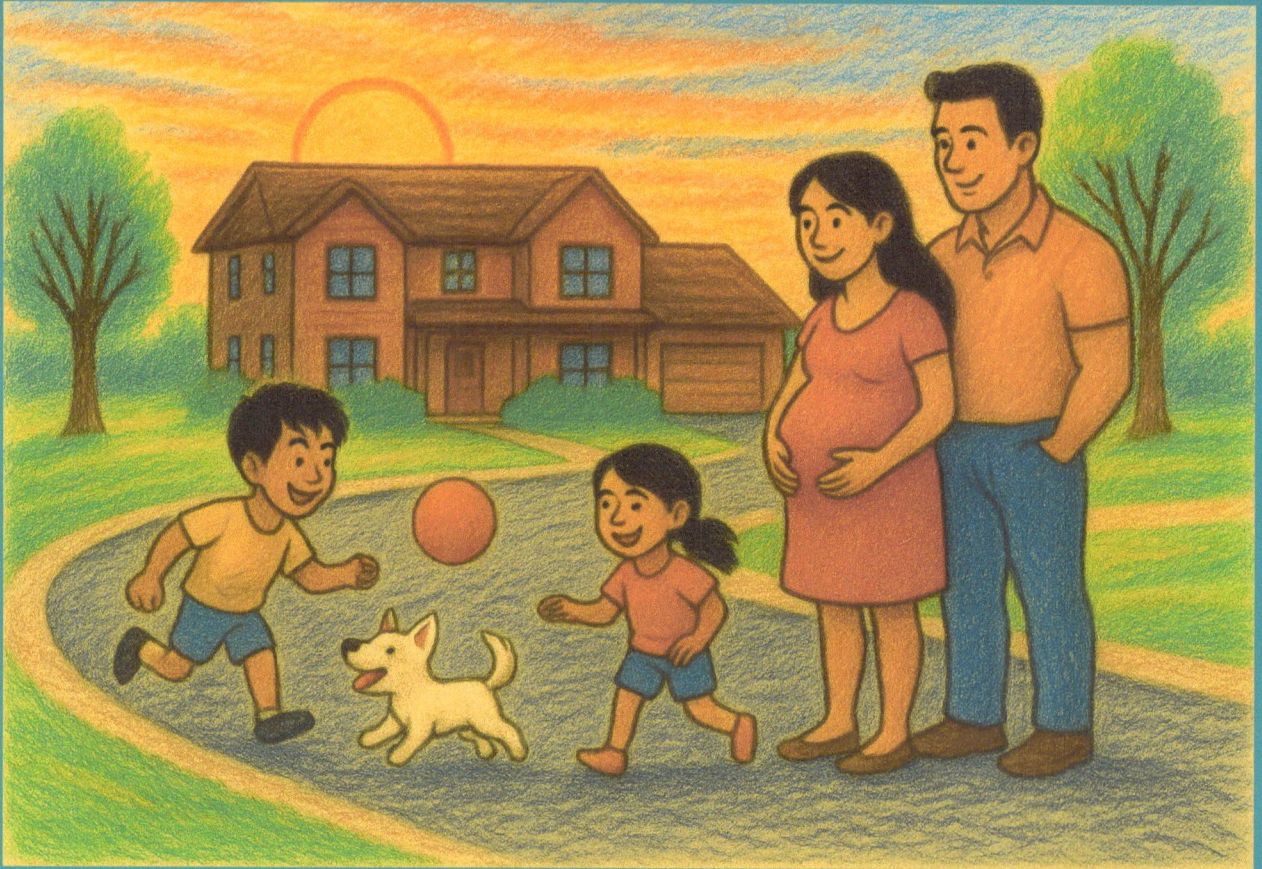

Two sweet kiddos with one on the way, working husband and wife.

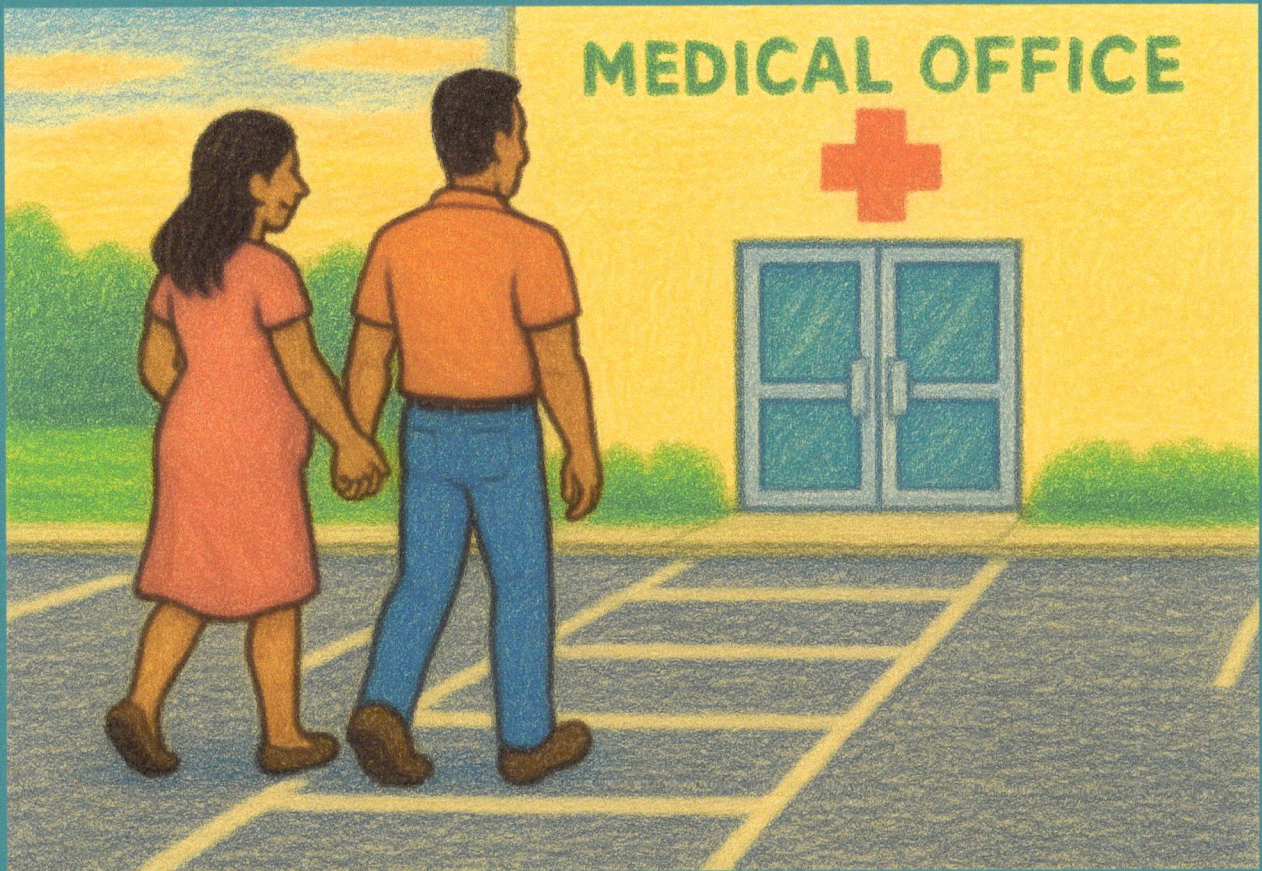

We loved our ultrasounds where we saw our baby grow,

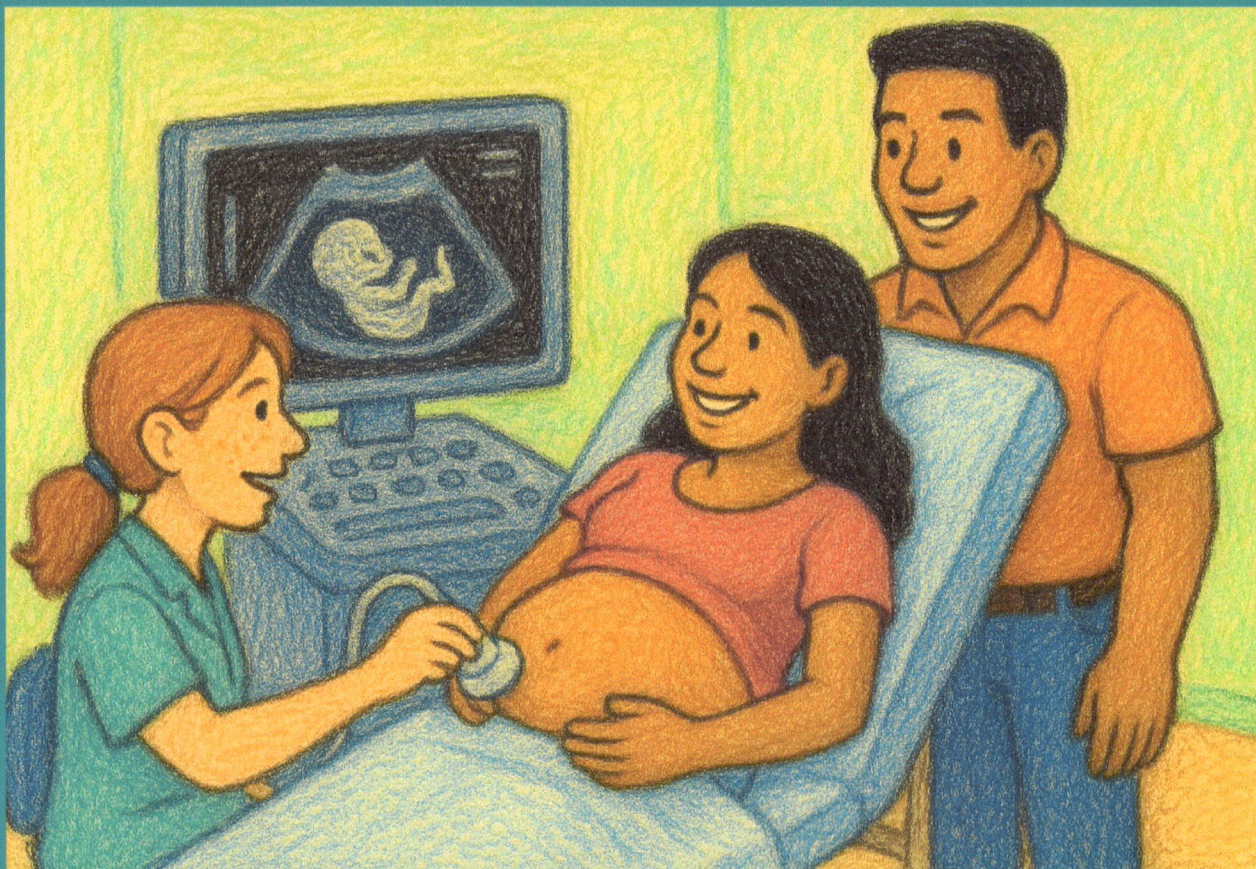

But the 20 week was our favorite for the 4D visualization show.

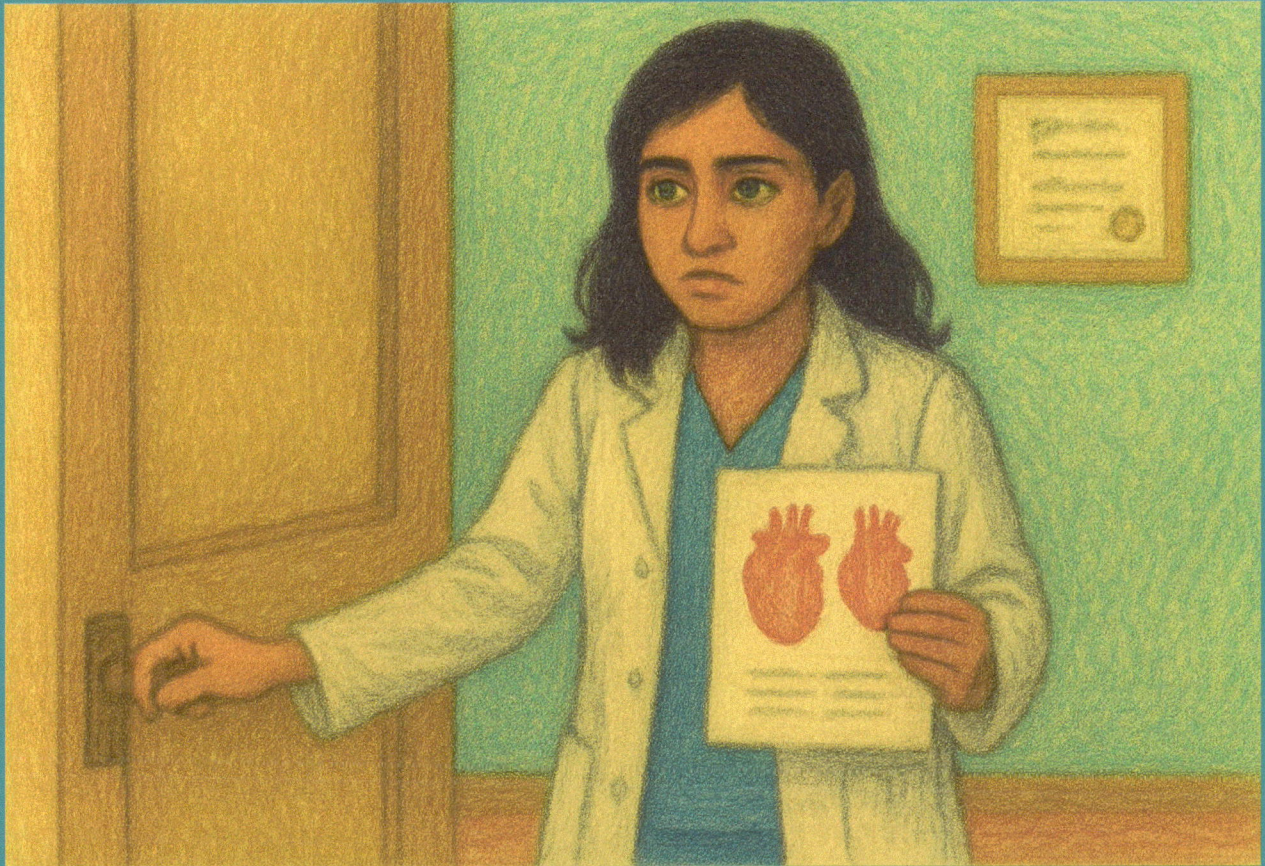

So when the room got quiet and the doctor sat down,

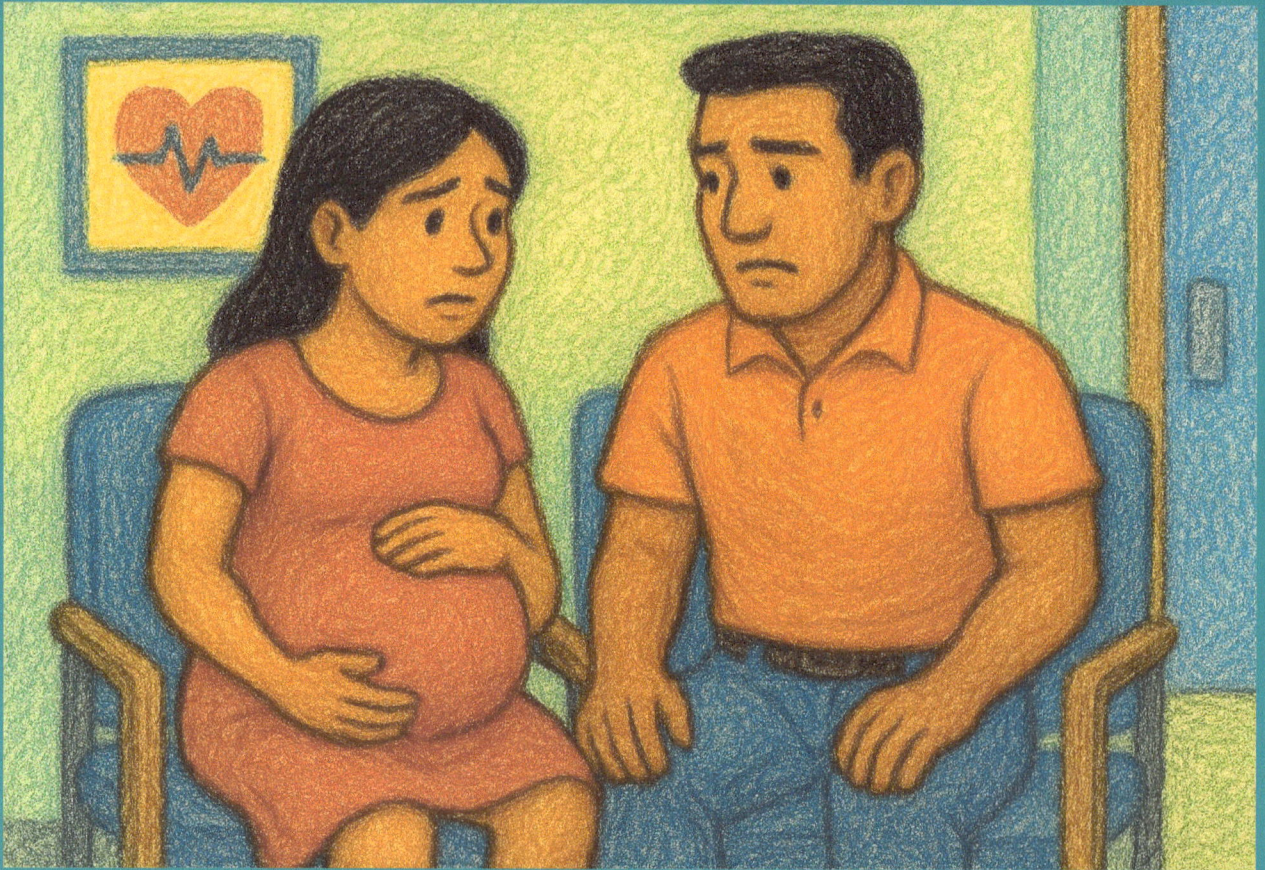

Our smiles and excitement turned to nervous frowns.

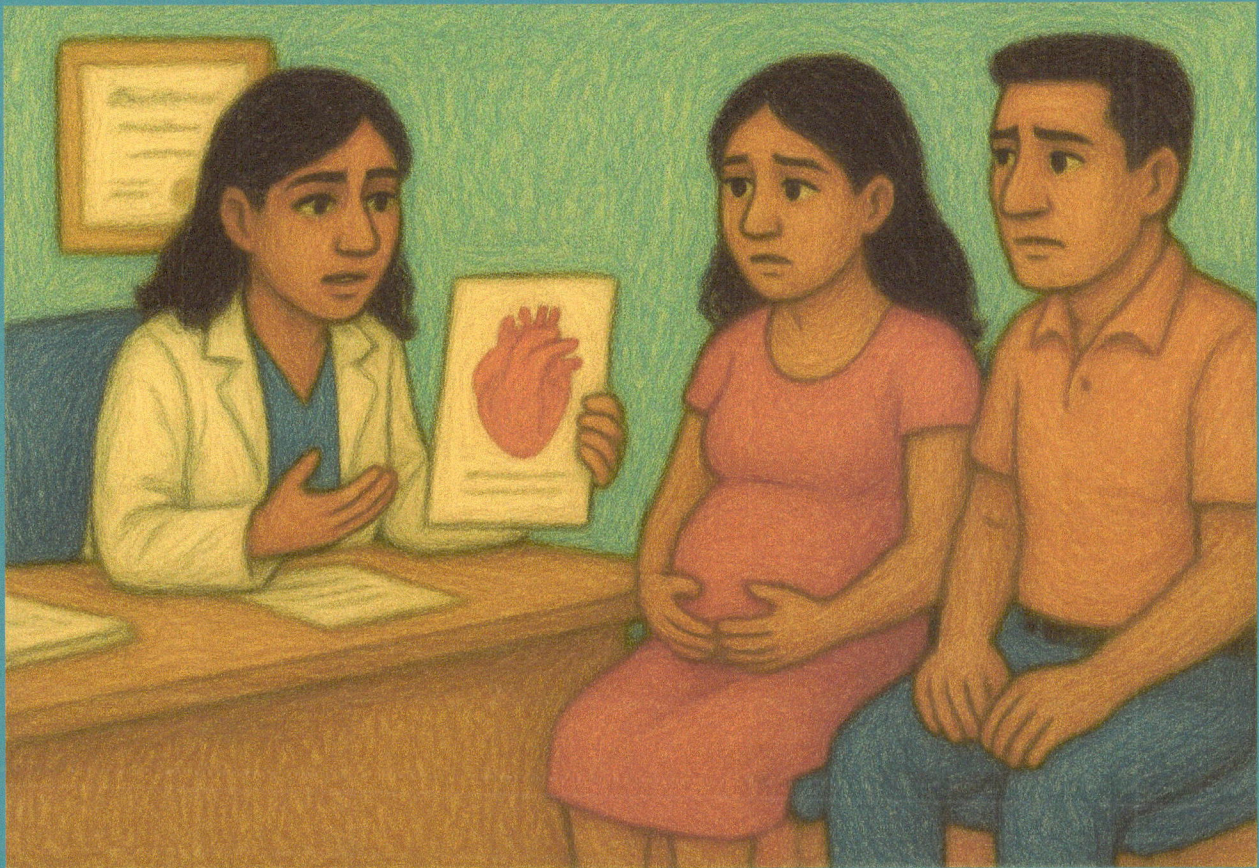

Your baby has half a heart, we're not sure why or how,

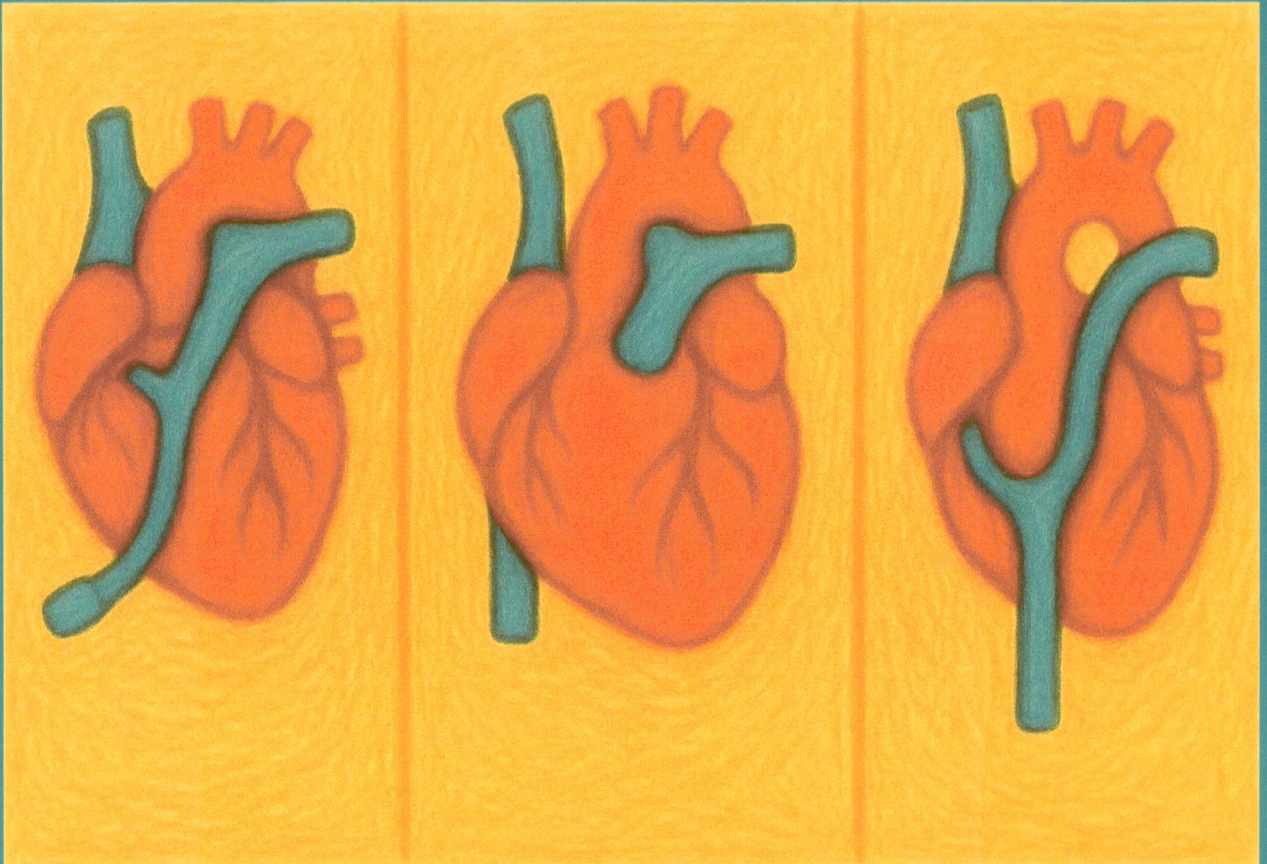

There will be open heart surgeries, what do you want to do now?

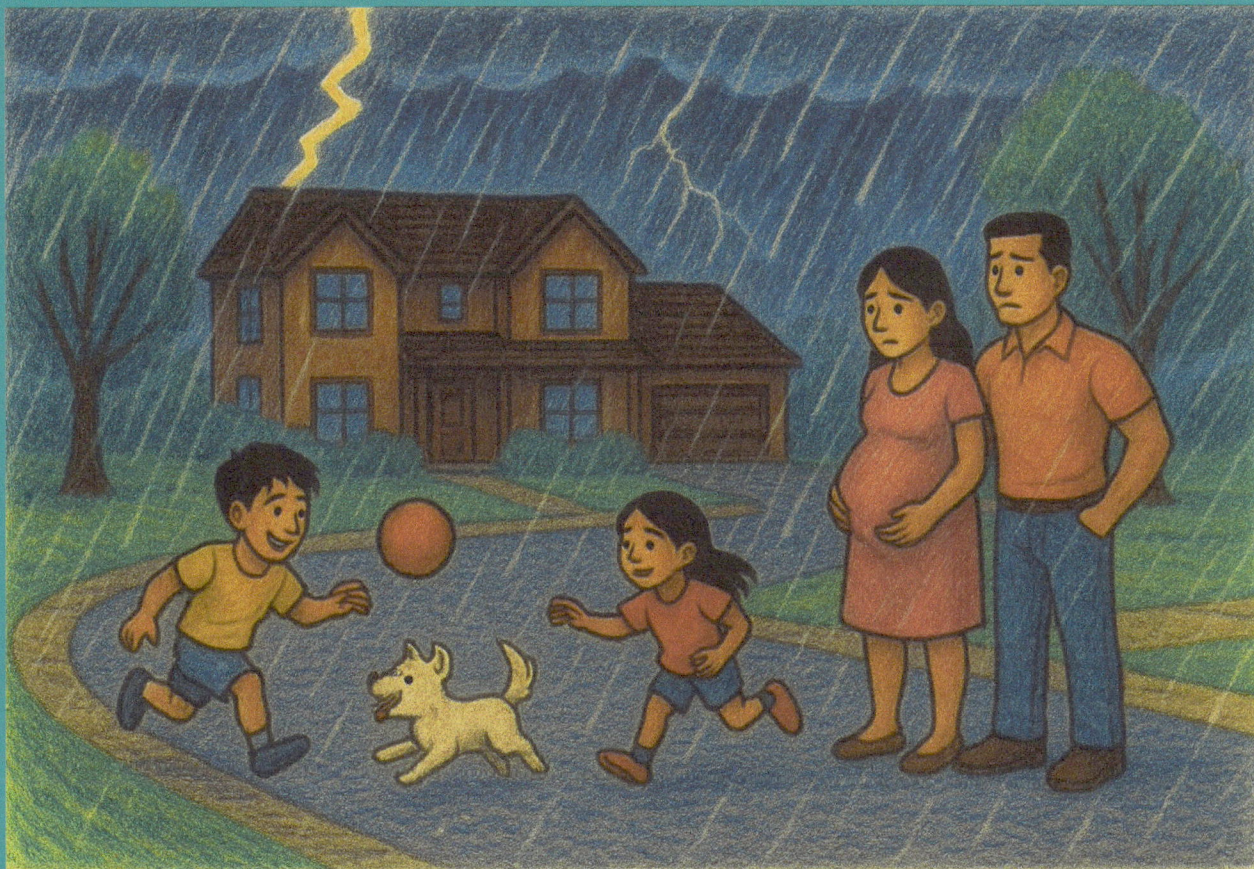

In a moment our world was shattered, like stopping mid-dance,

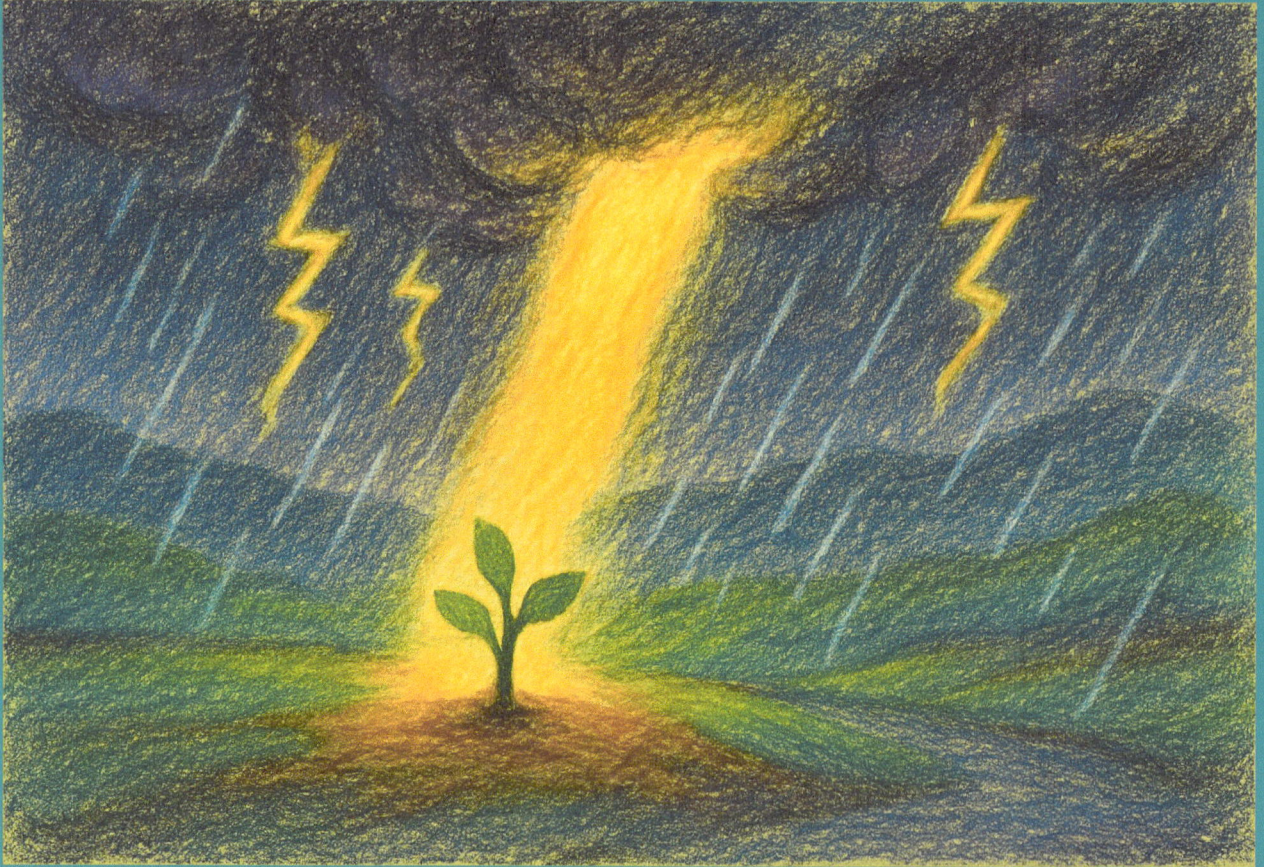

The medical team told us it would be hard, but he had a chance.

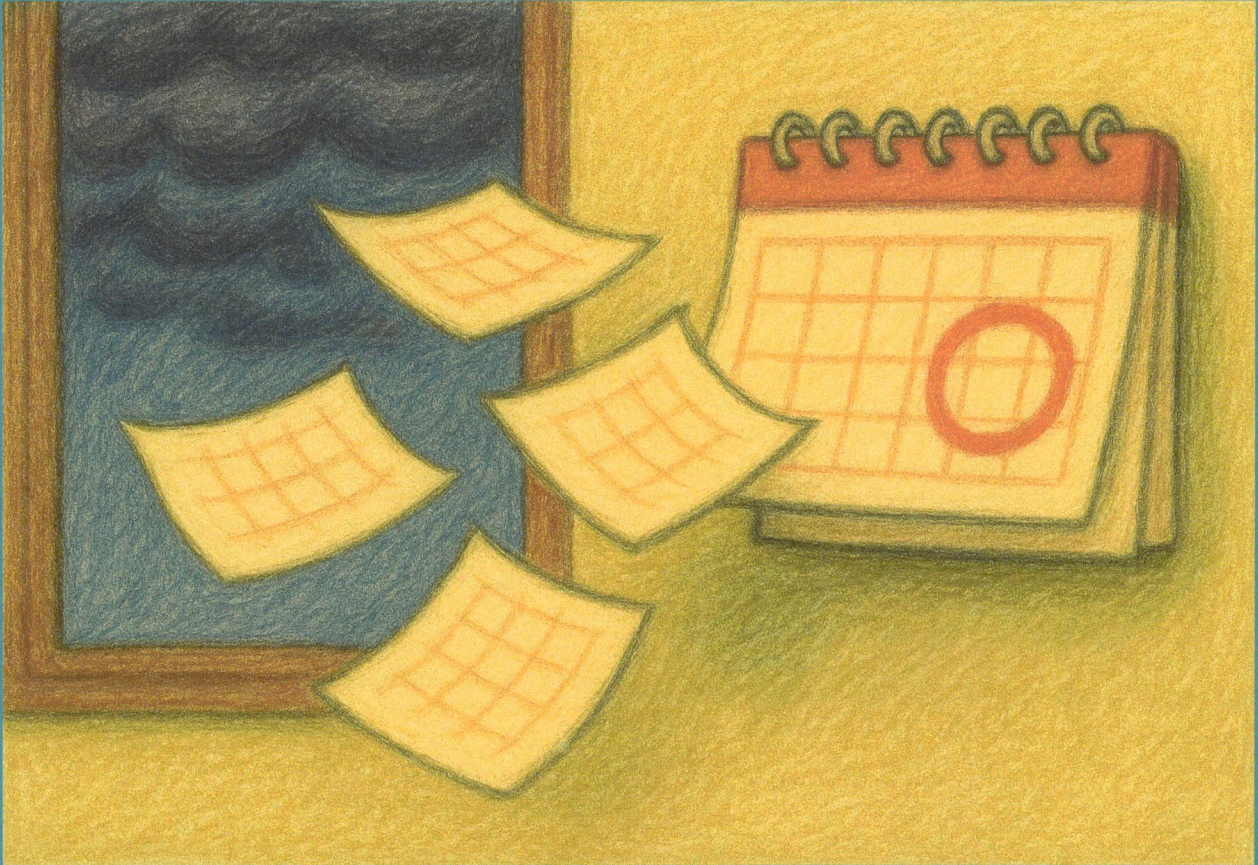

We planned and worried for his special birth day,

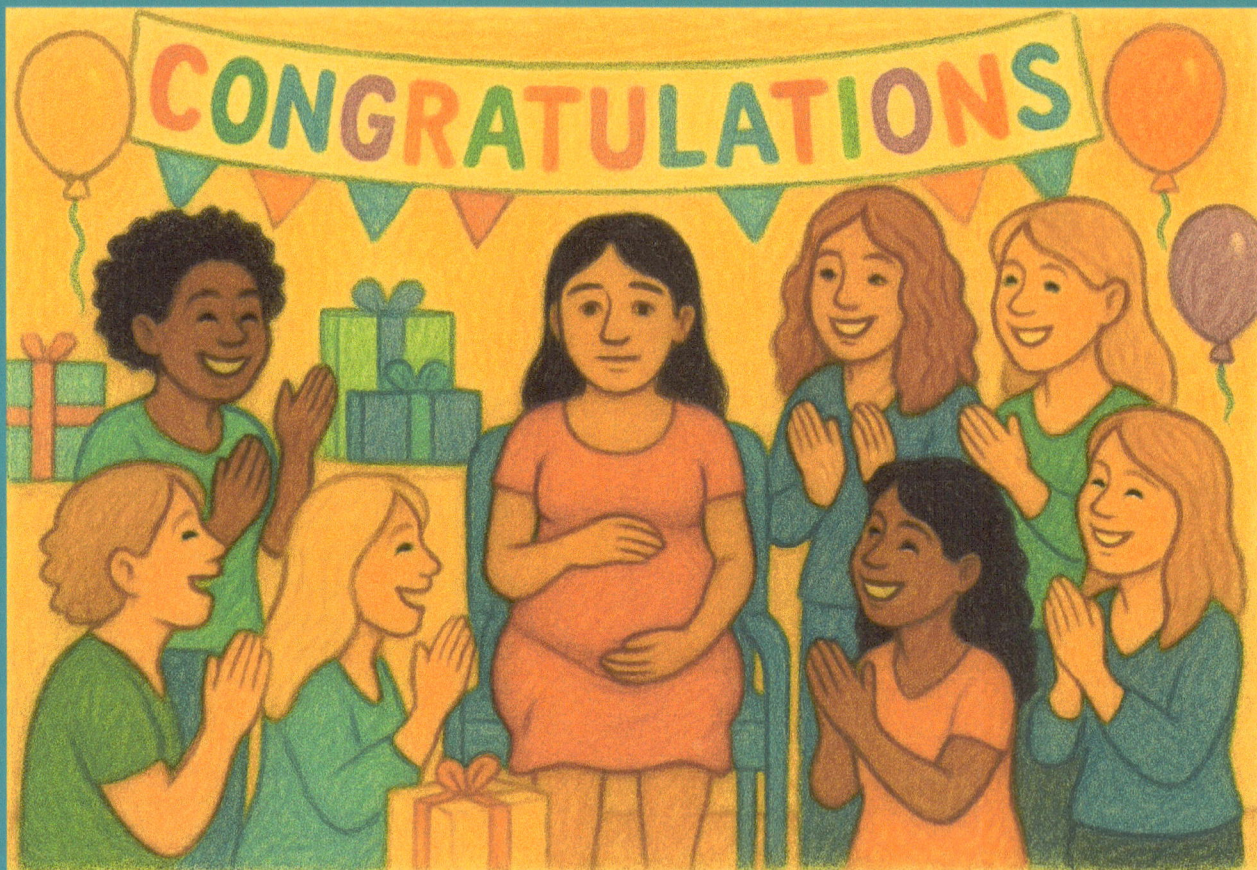

Many said, "Can't wait until he's born!" We didn't know what to say.

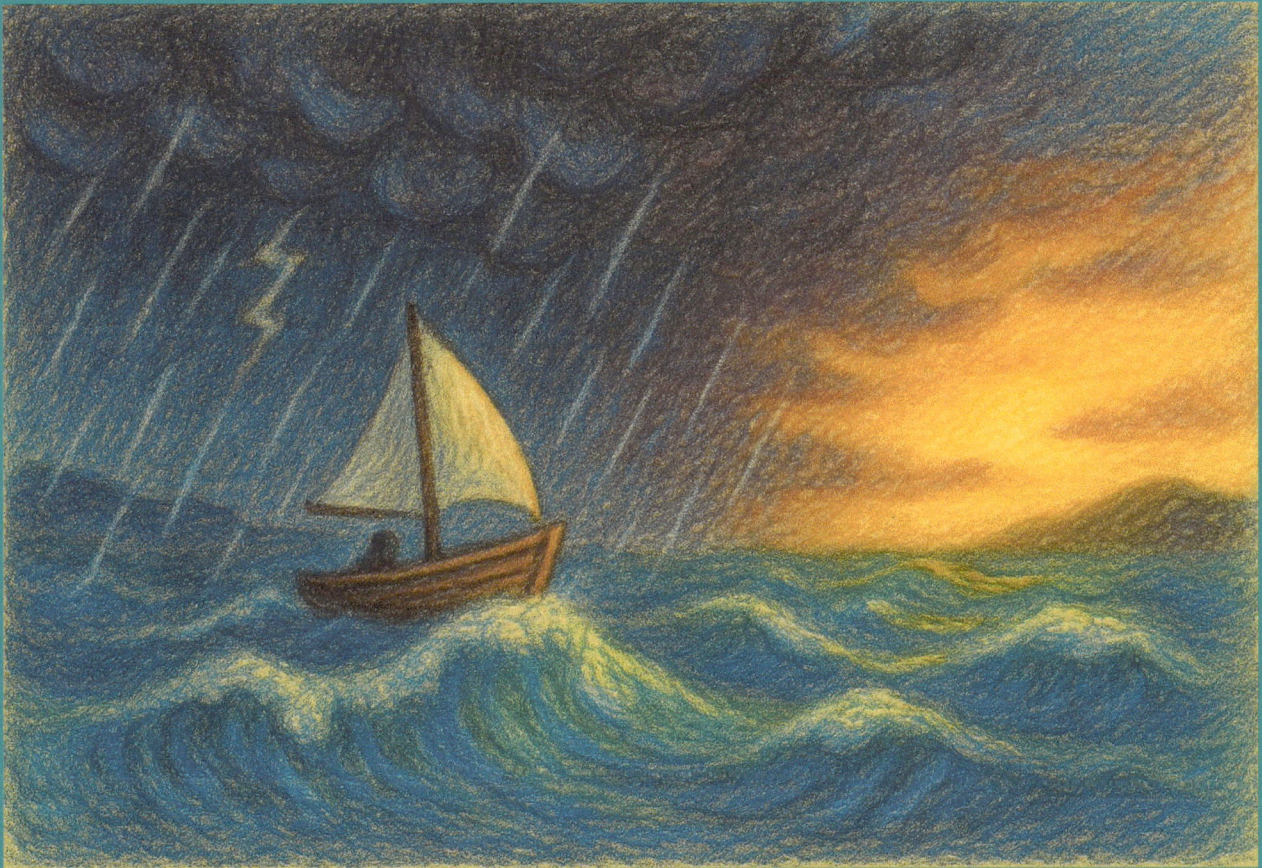

But we knew there was a plan, something we couldn't explain,

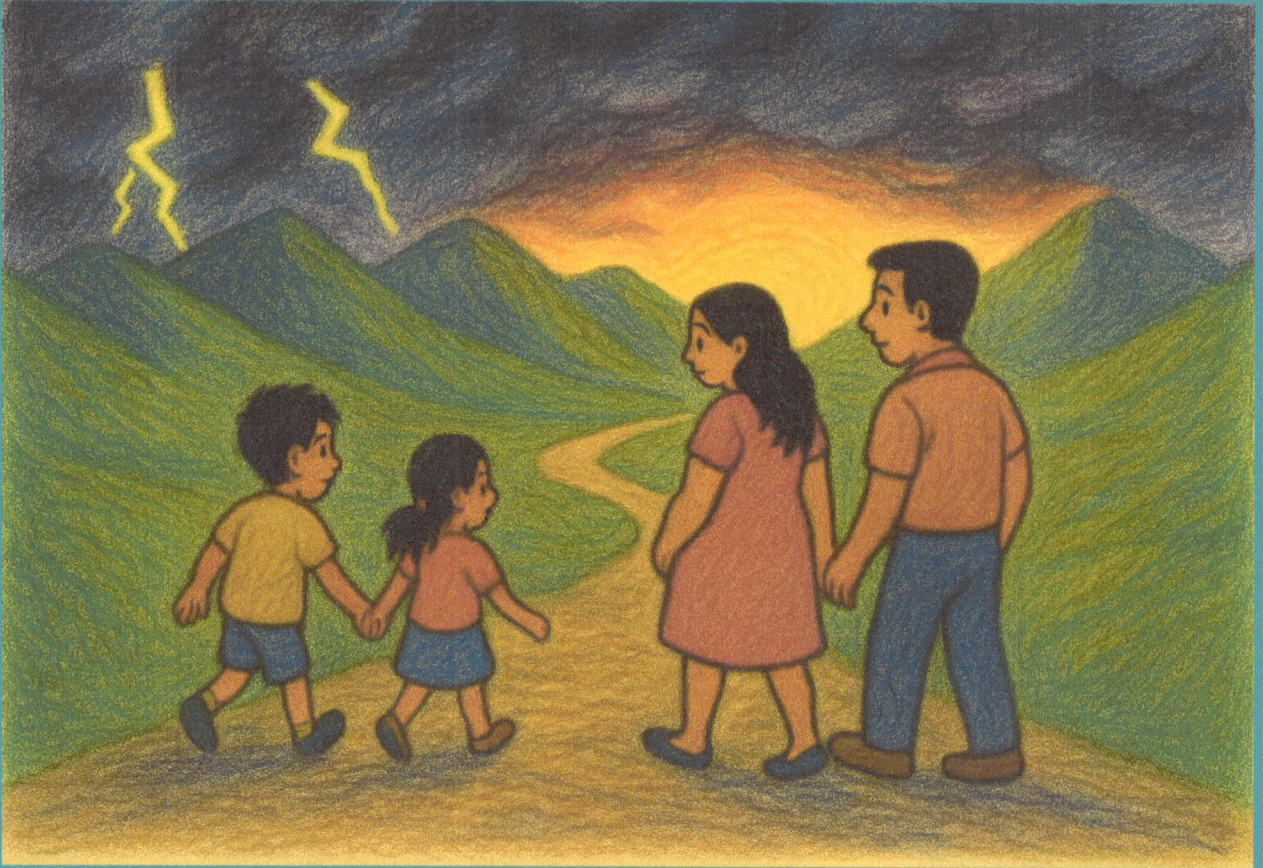

His life would be hard, but purpose in the pain.

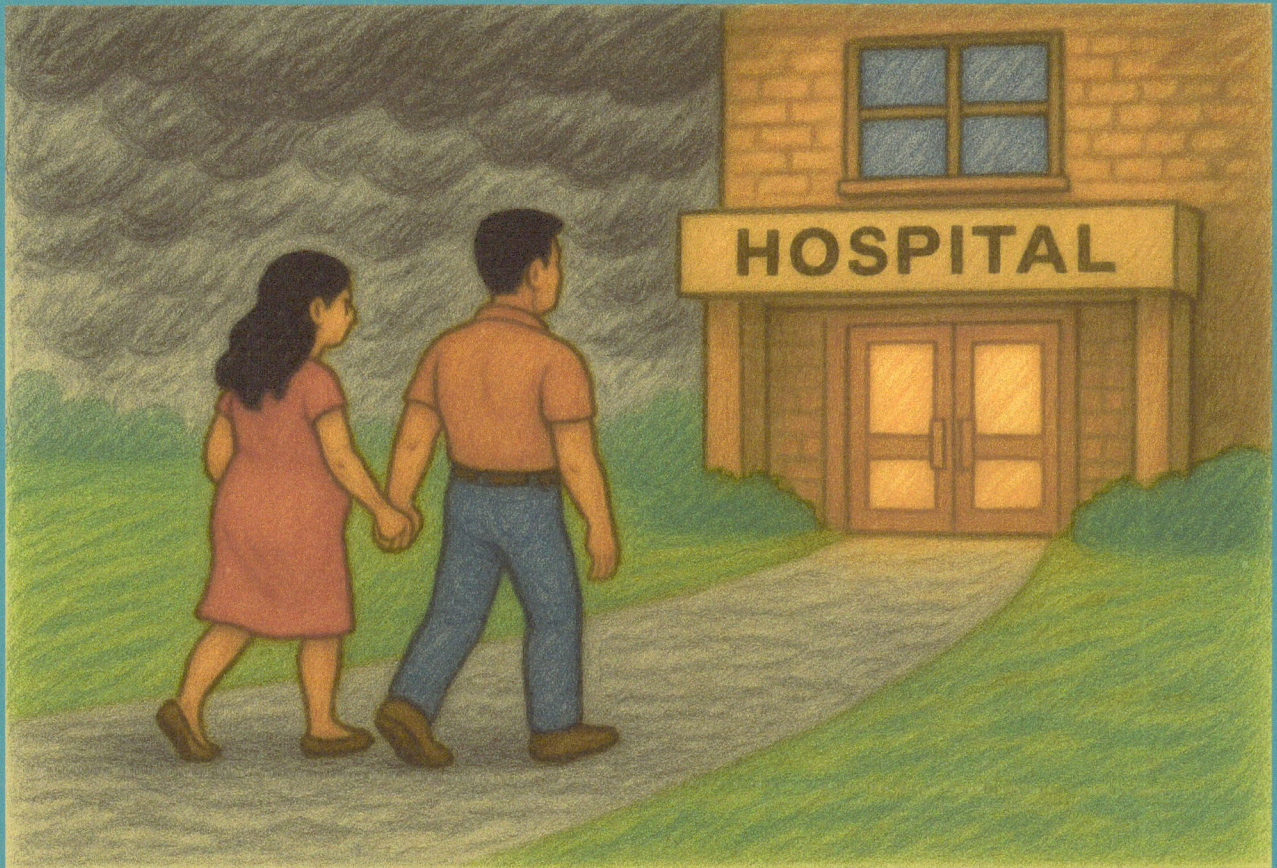

We went to the hospital, the day had finally come,

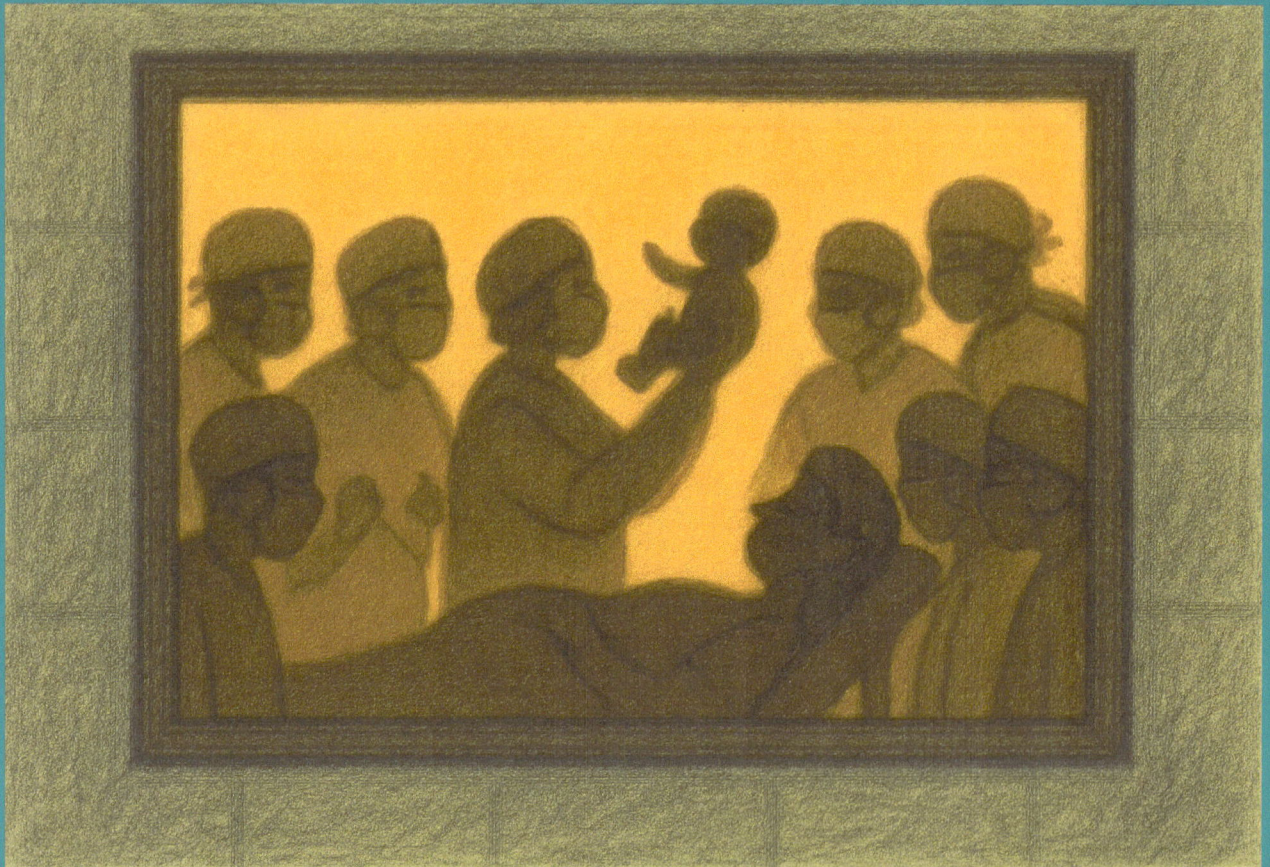

He was born blue and needed help, but his team got it done.

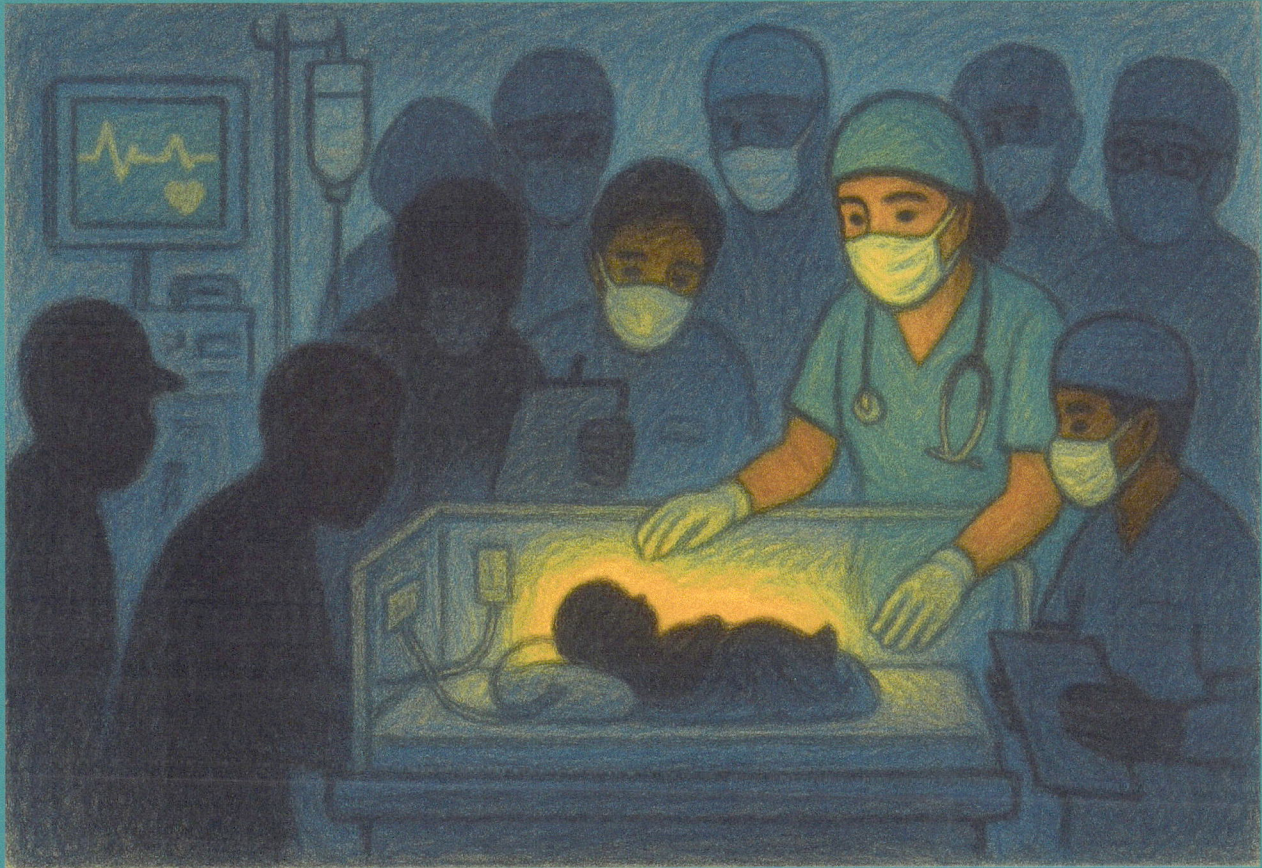

Part of a heart community, with a team of experts by our side,

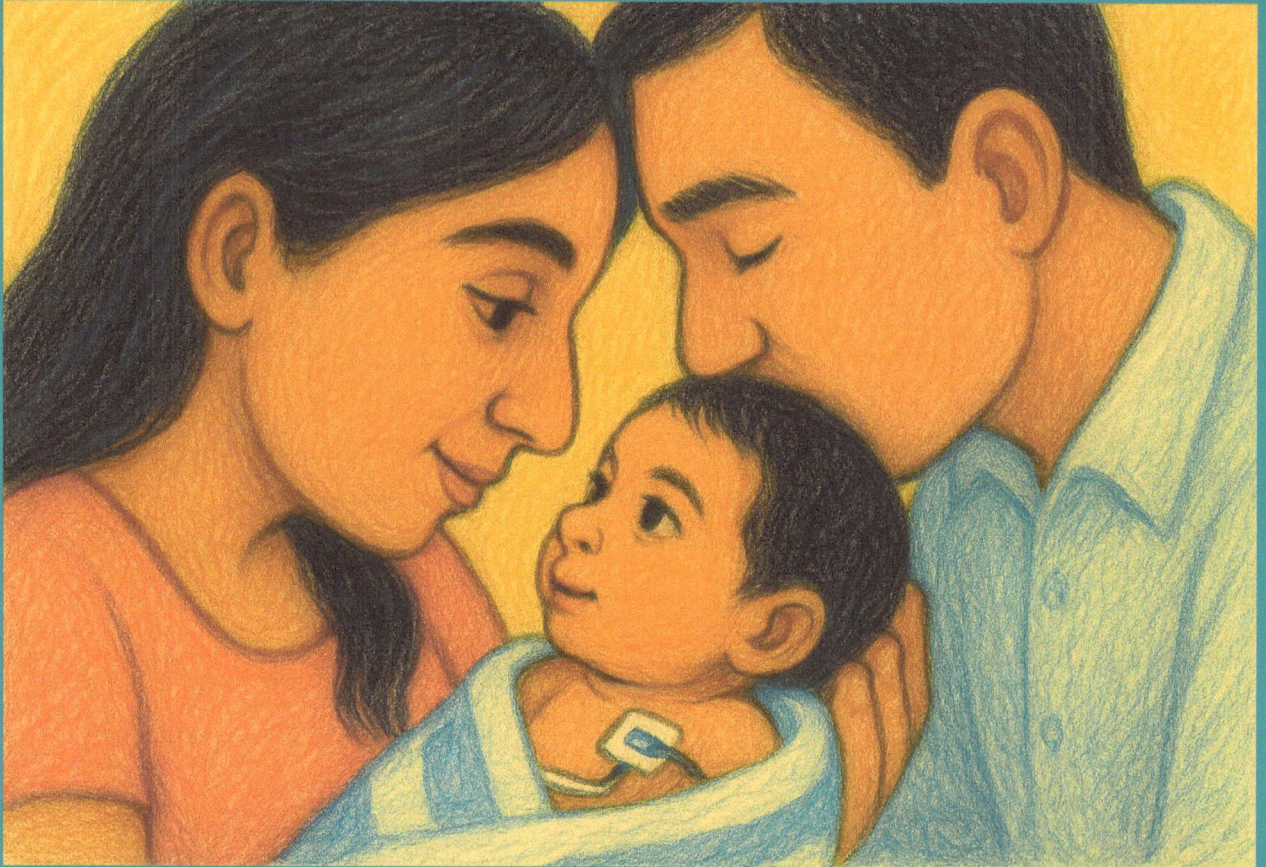

His heart frail, eyes perfect, inviting us on his heart ride.

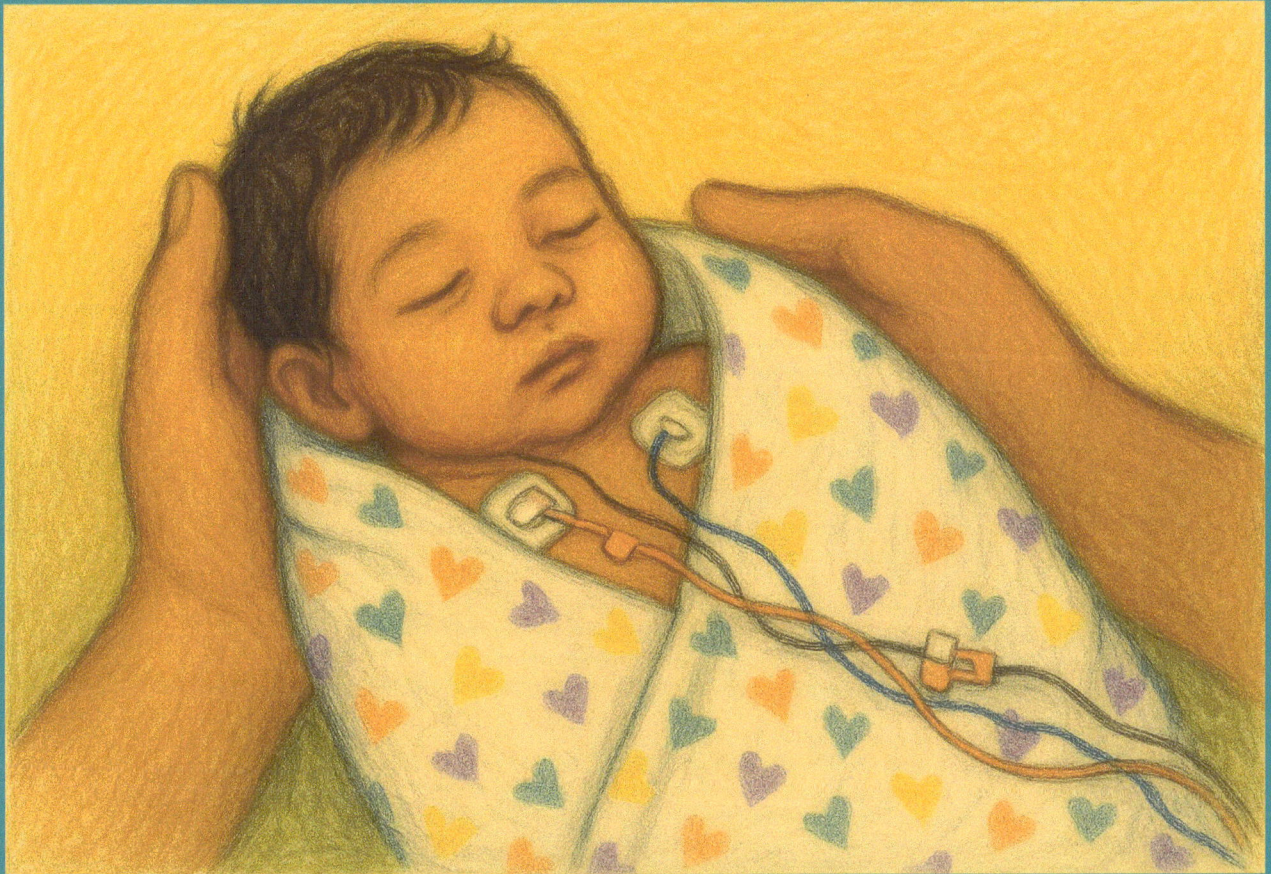

The first surgery was the hardest, his heart and body were so small,

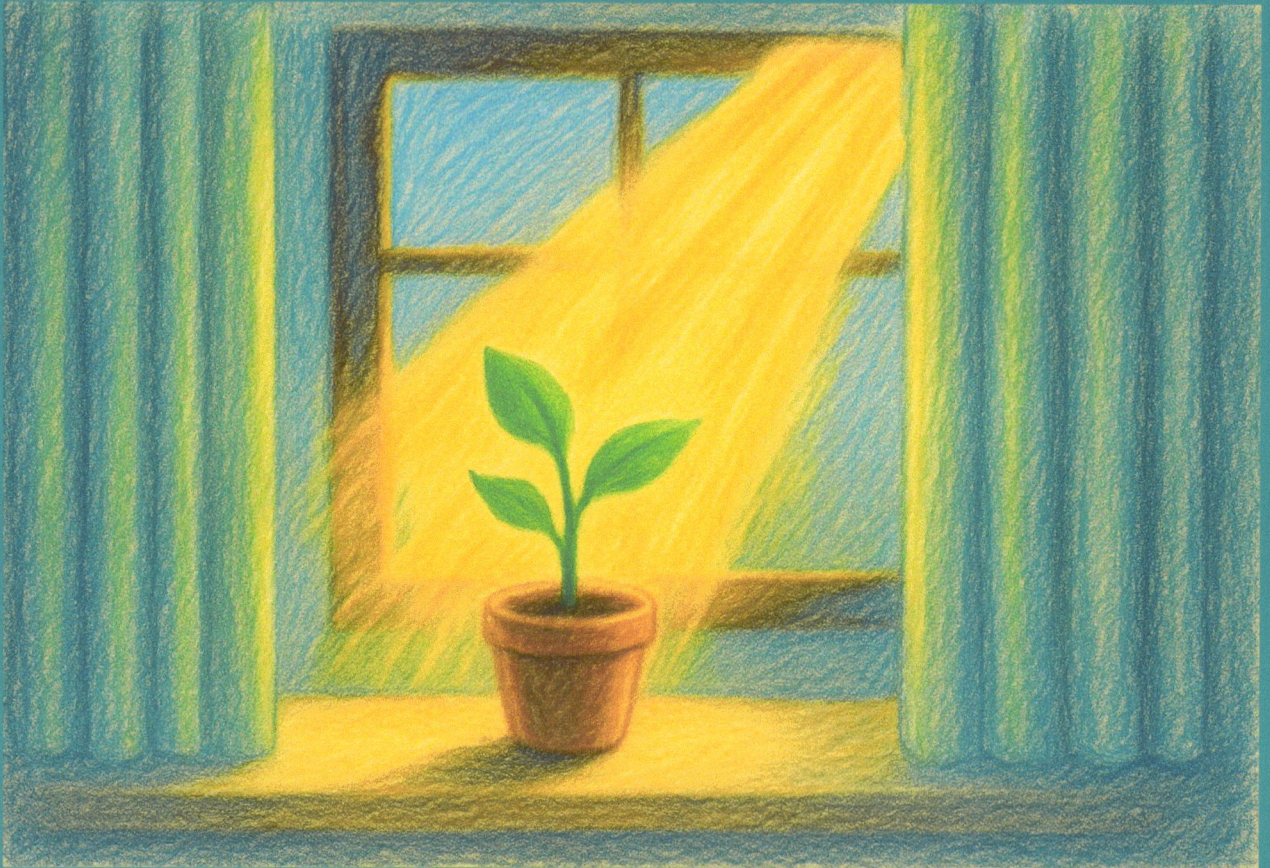

But he taught us to have faith through it all.

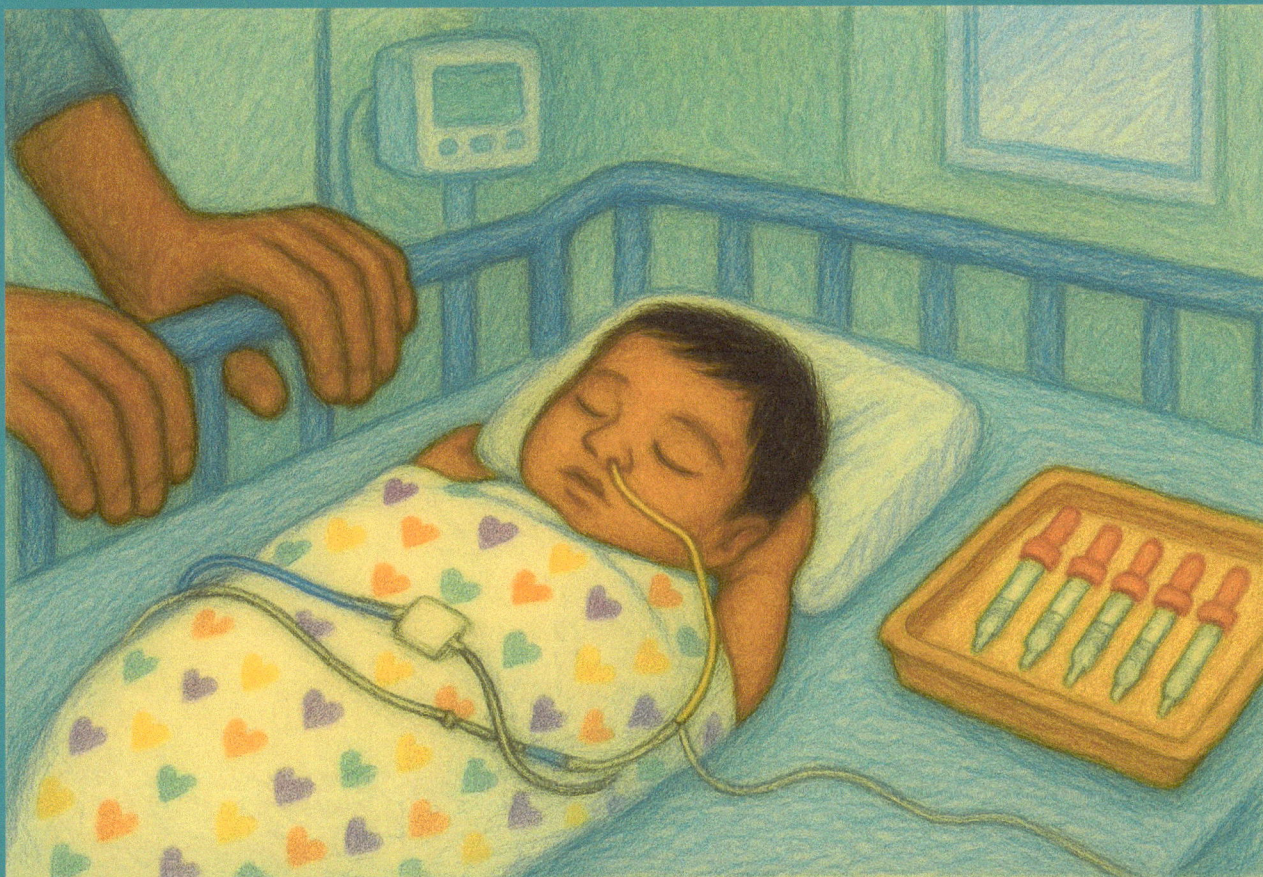

We learned about feeding, medications, so many medical terms.

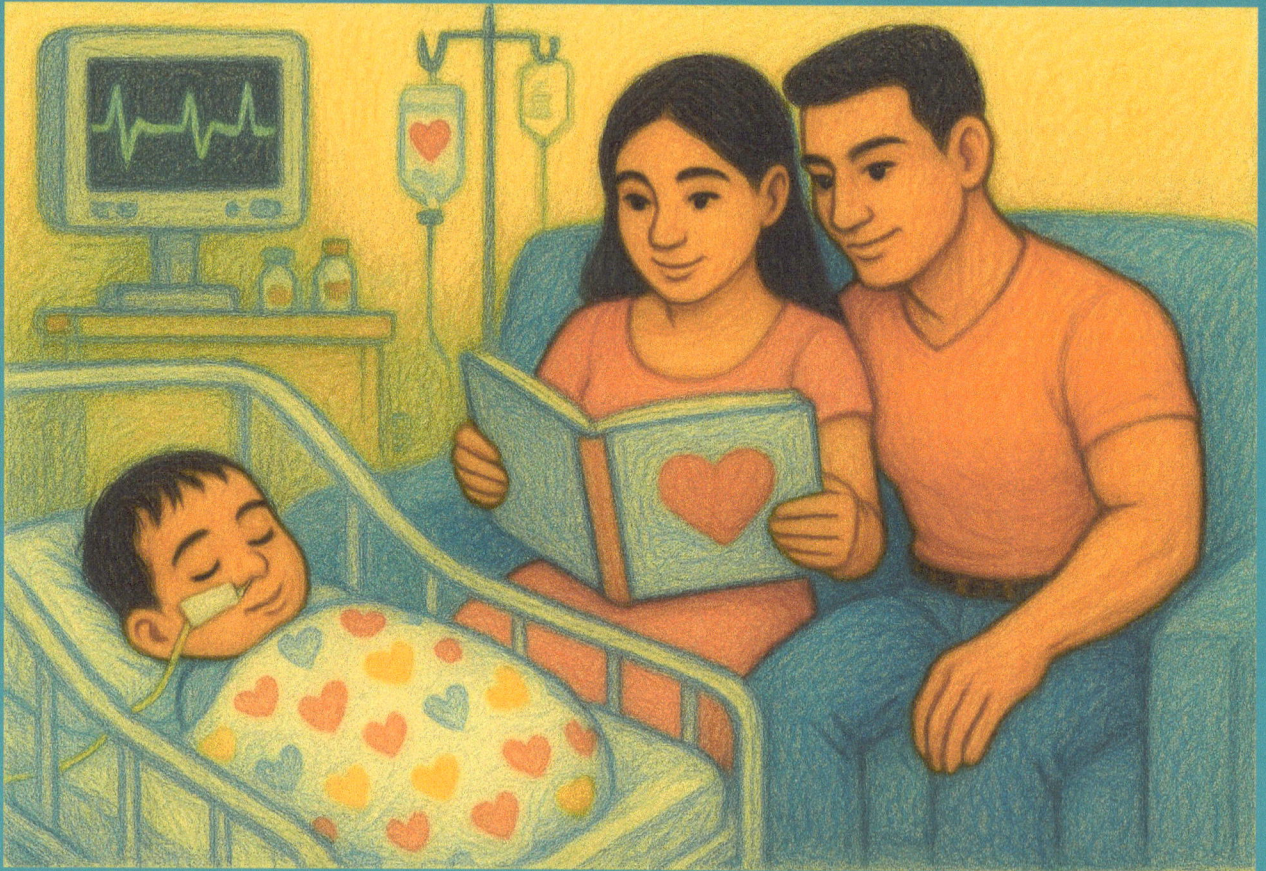

But his love was so great, patiently he helped us learn.

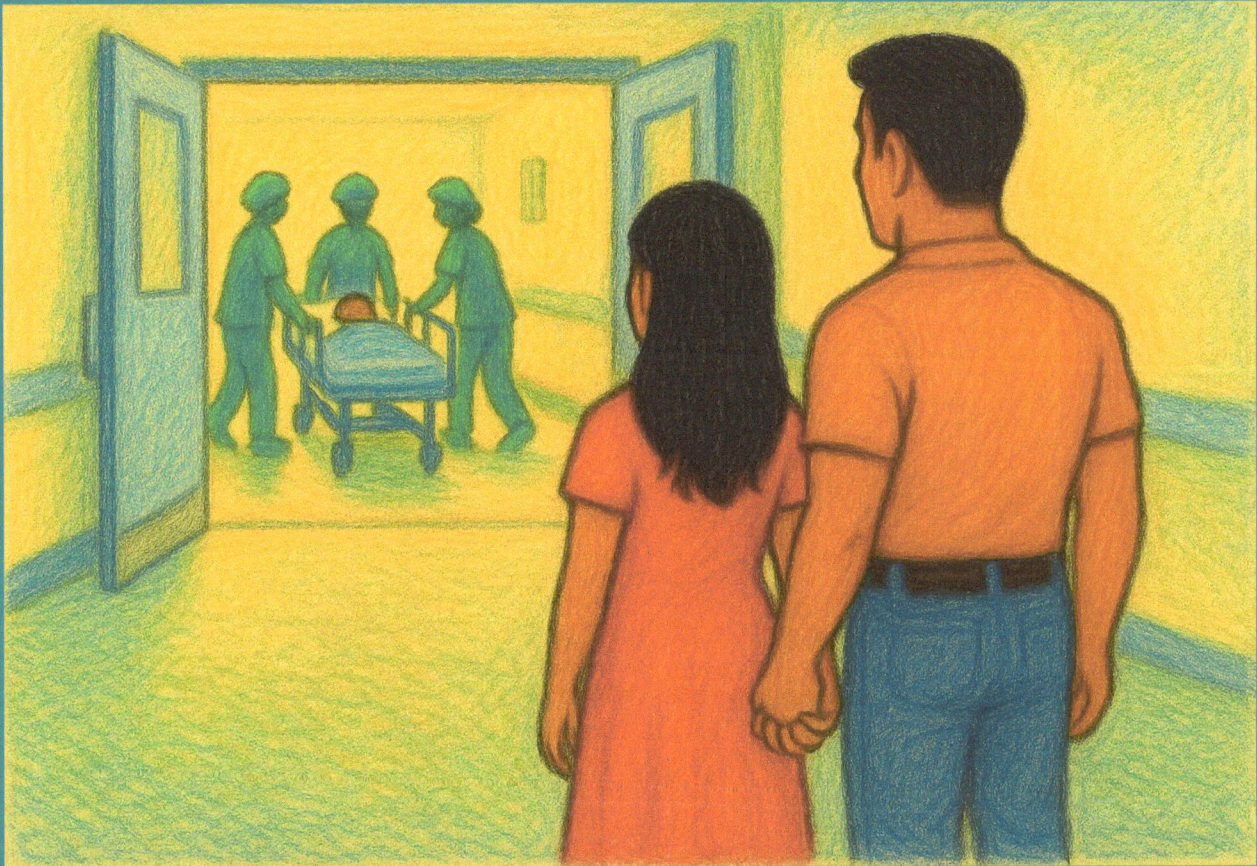

The second surgery was also tough, but knew more what to expect,

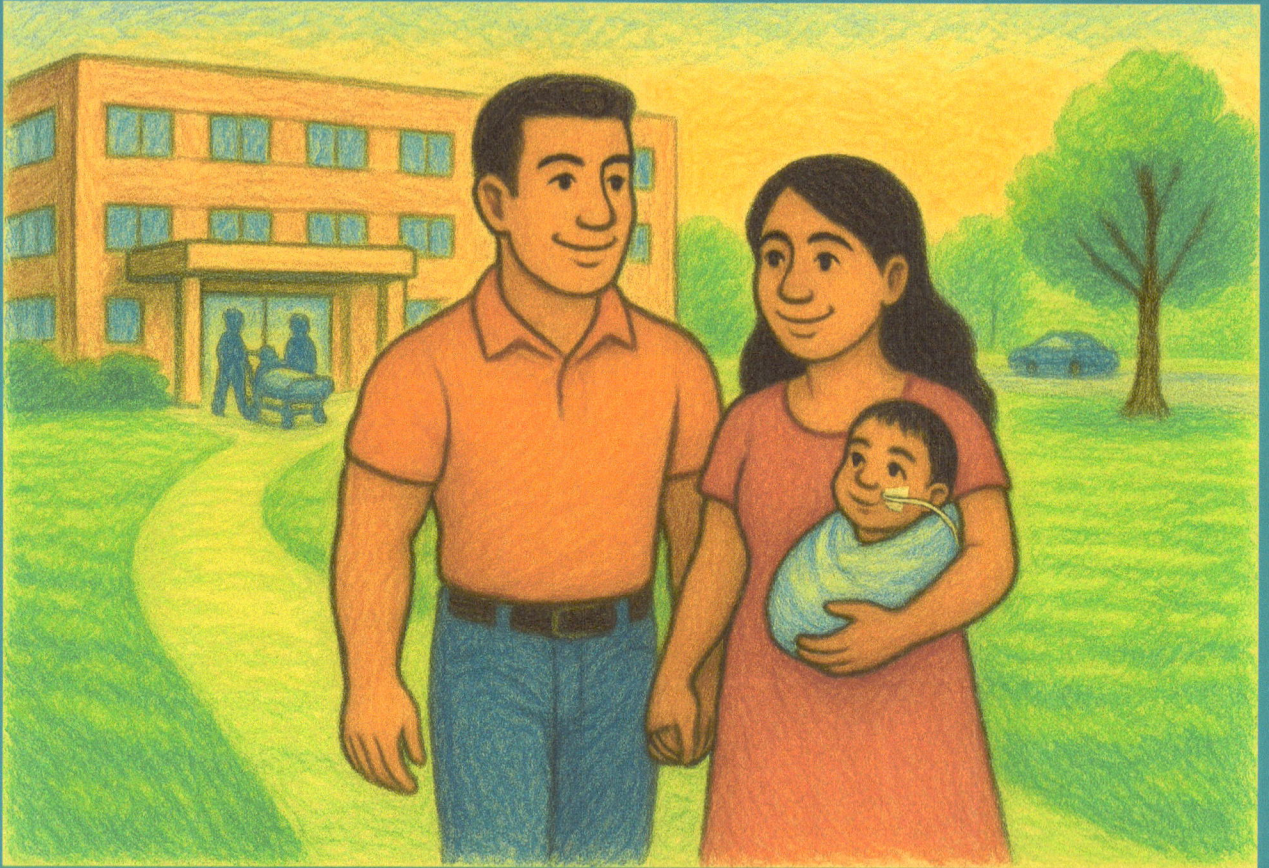

We faced new challenges, but the path home was more direct.

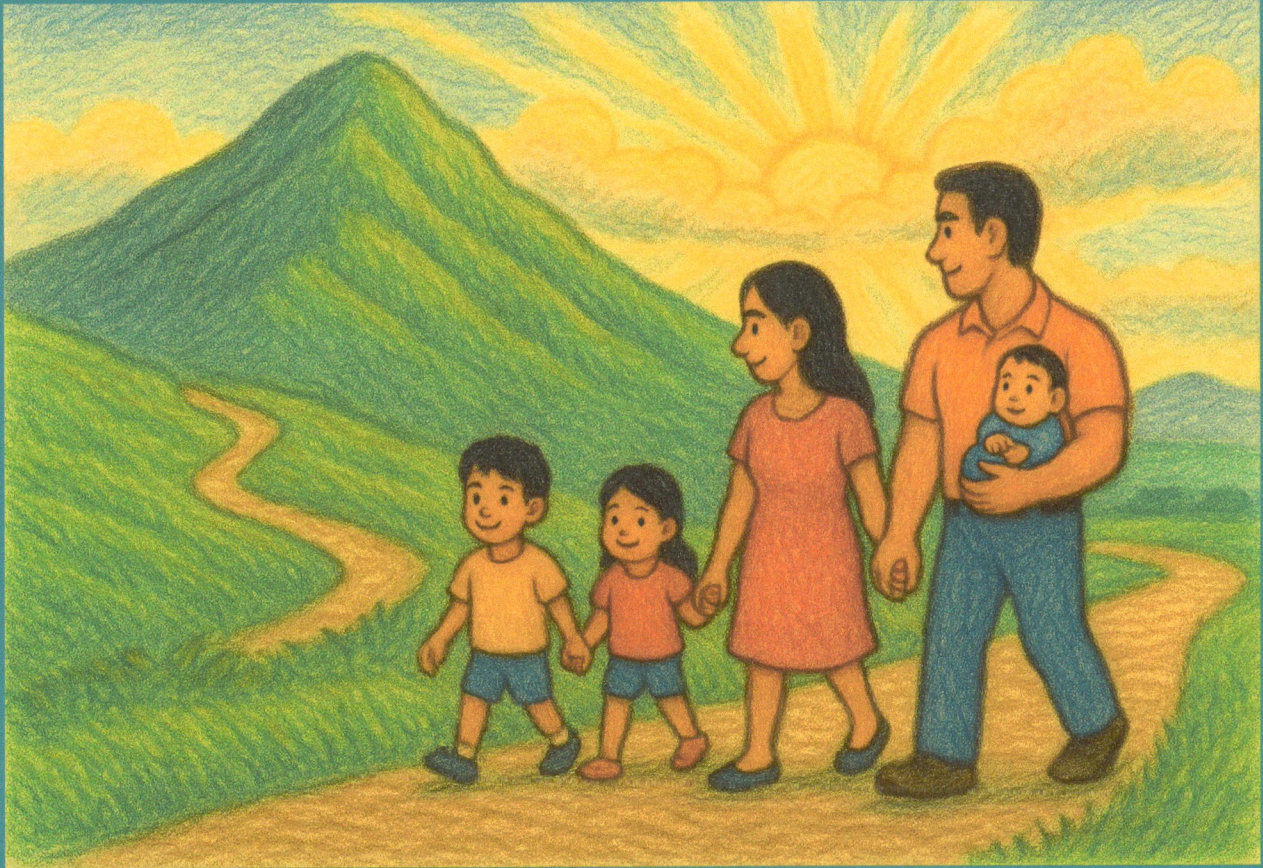

The journey of our special baby has been more than we thought.

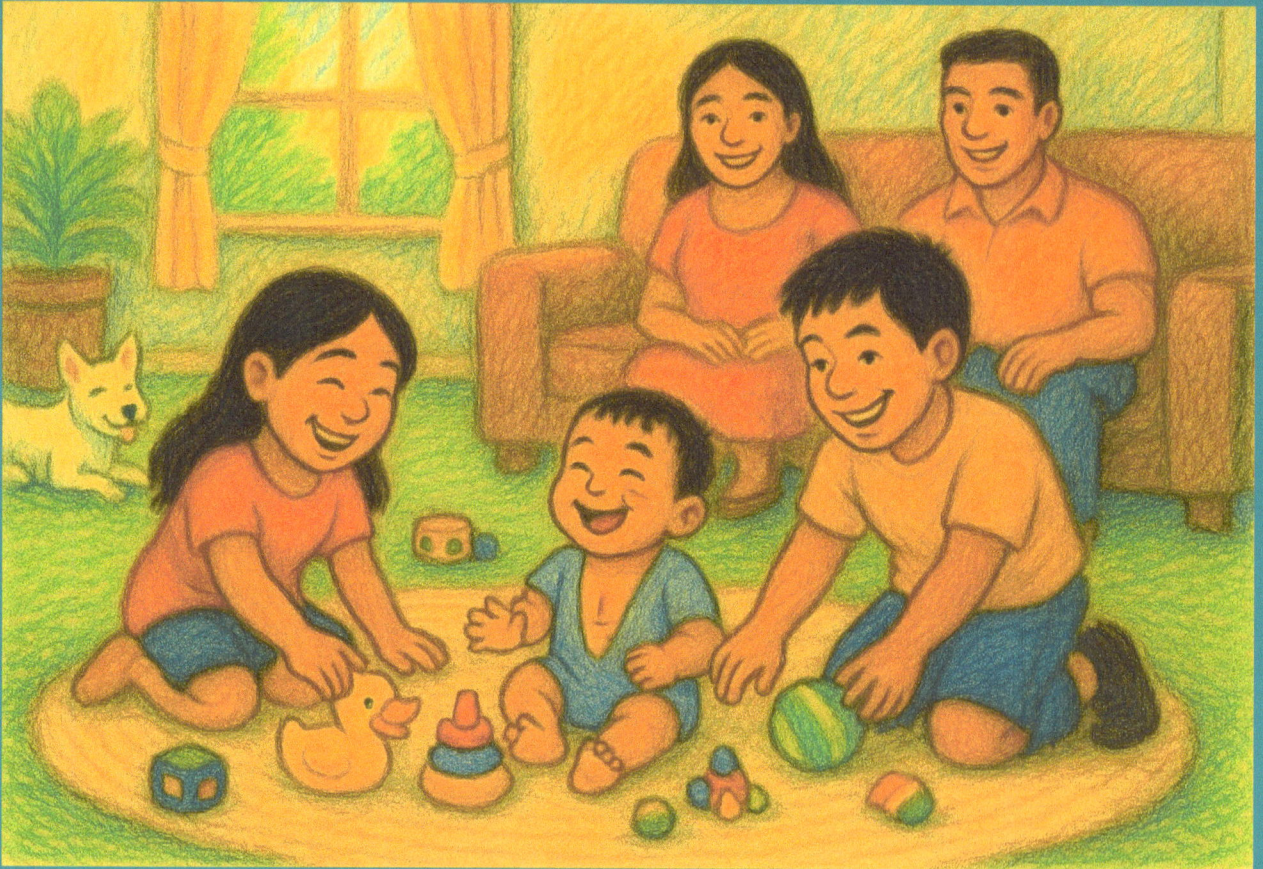

But seeing his face, hearing his laugh, make us thankful we fought.

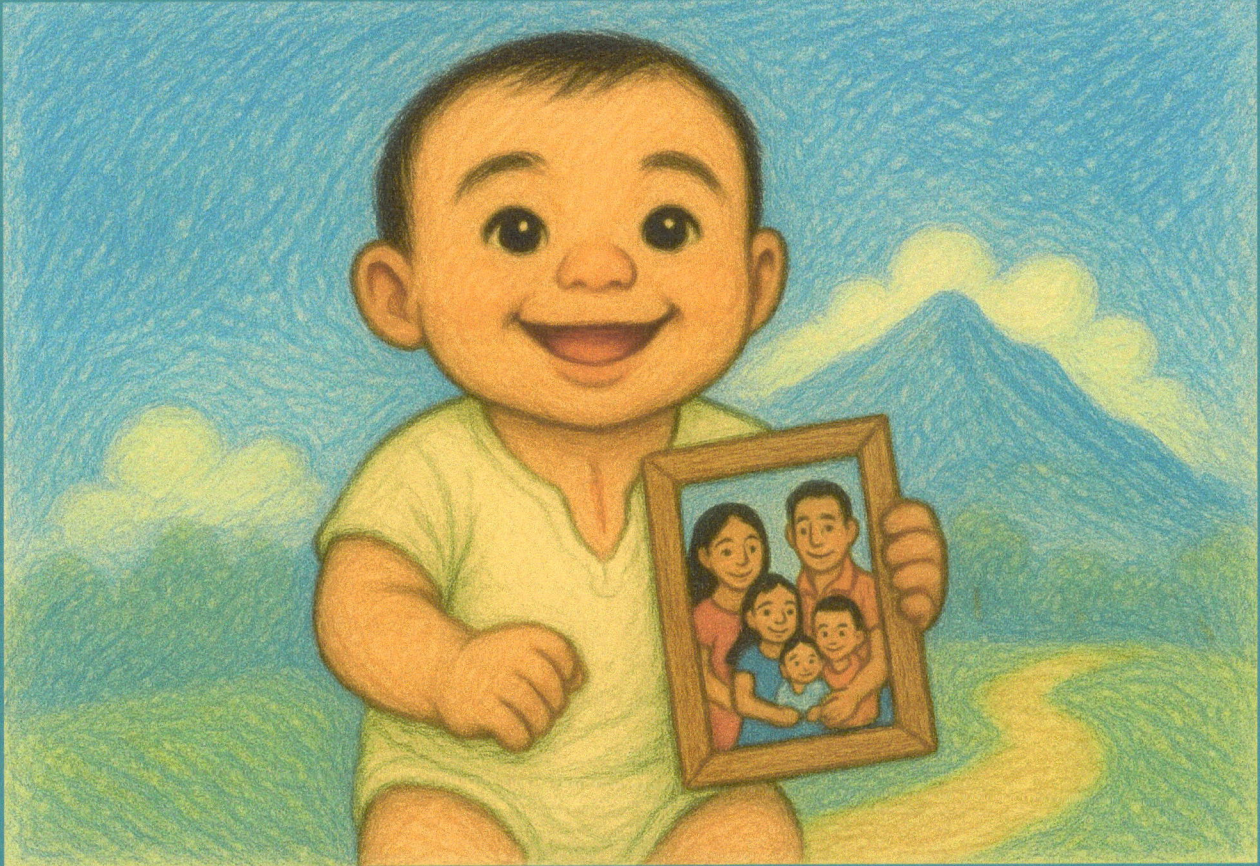

He is our warrior and we will continue to fight strong,

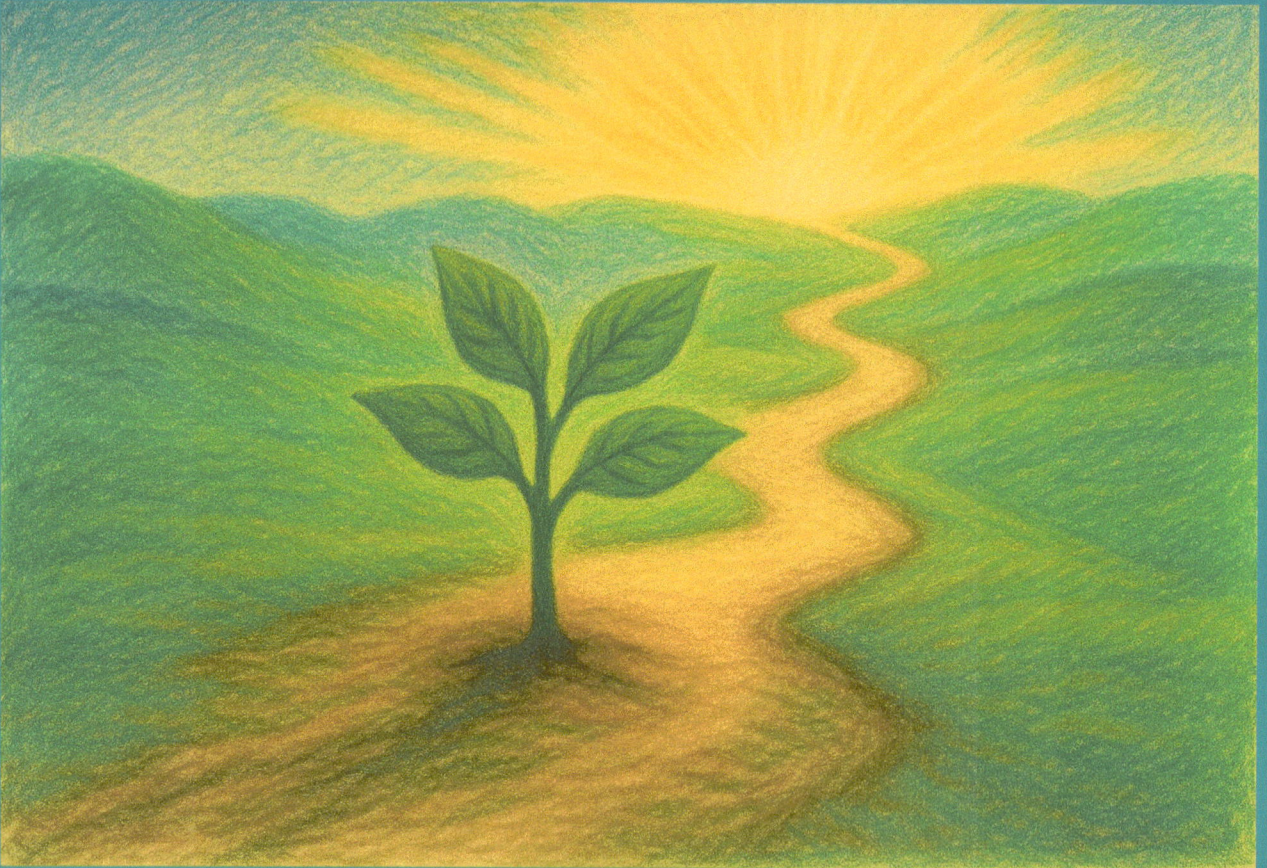

Through the painful, long journey we continue to walk along.

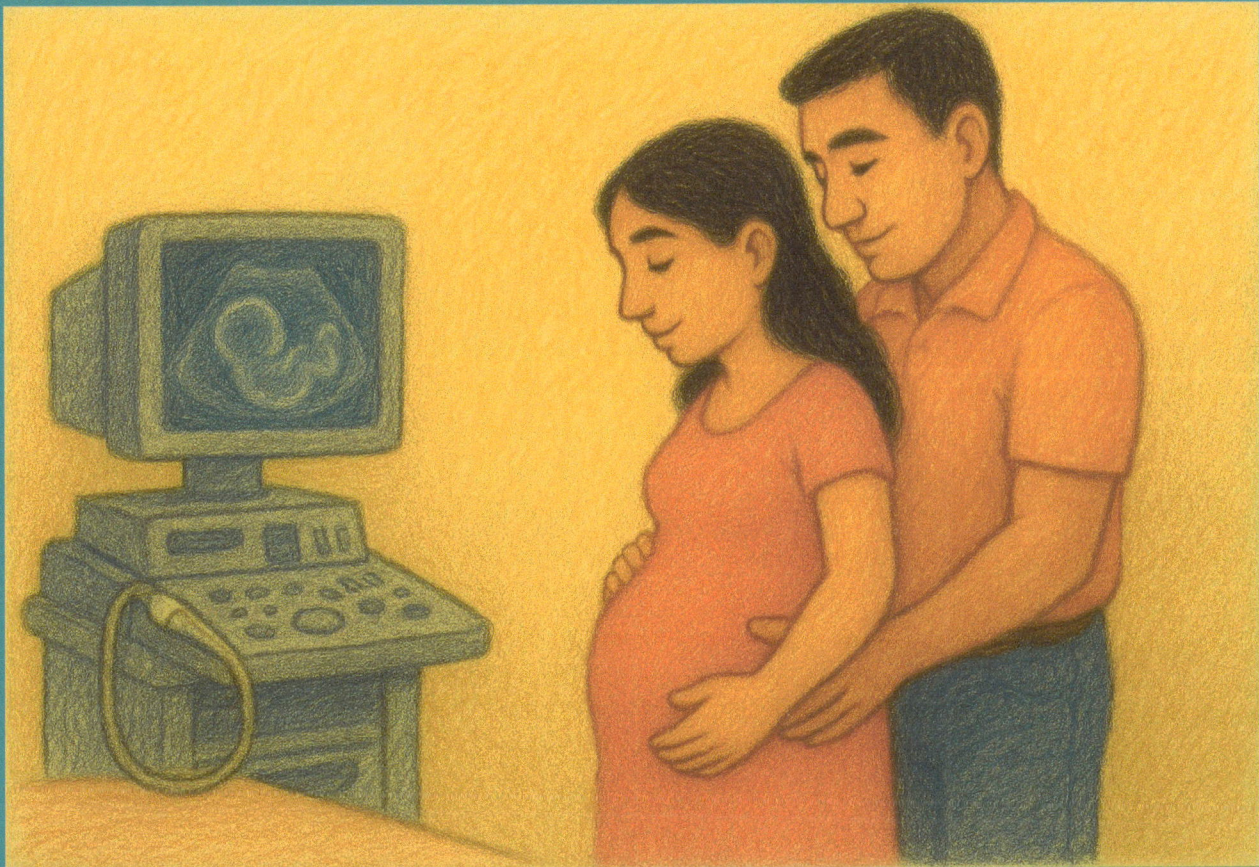

We did not know who he would be, who we would be,

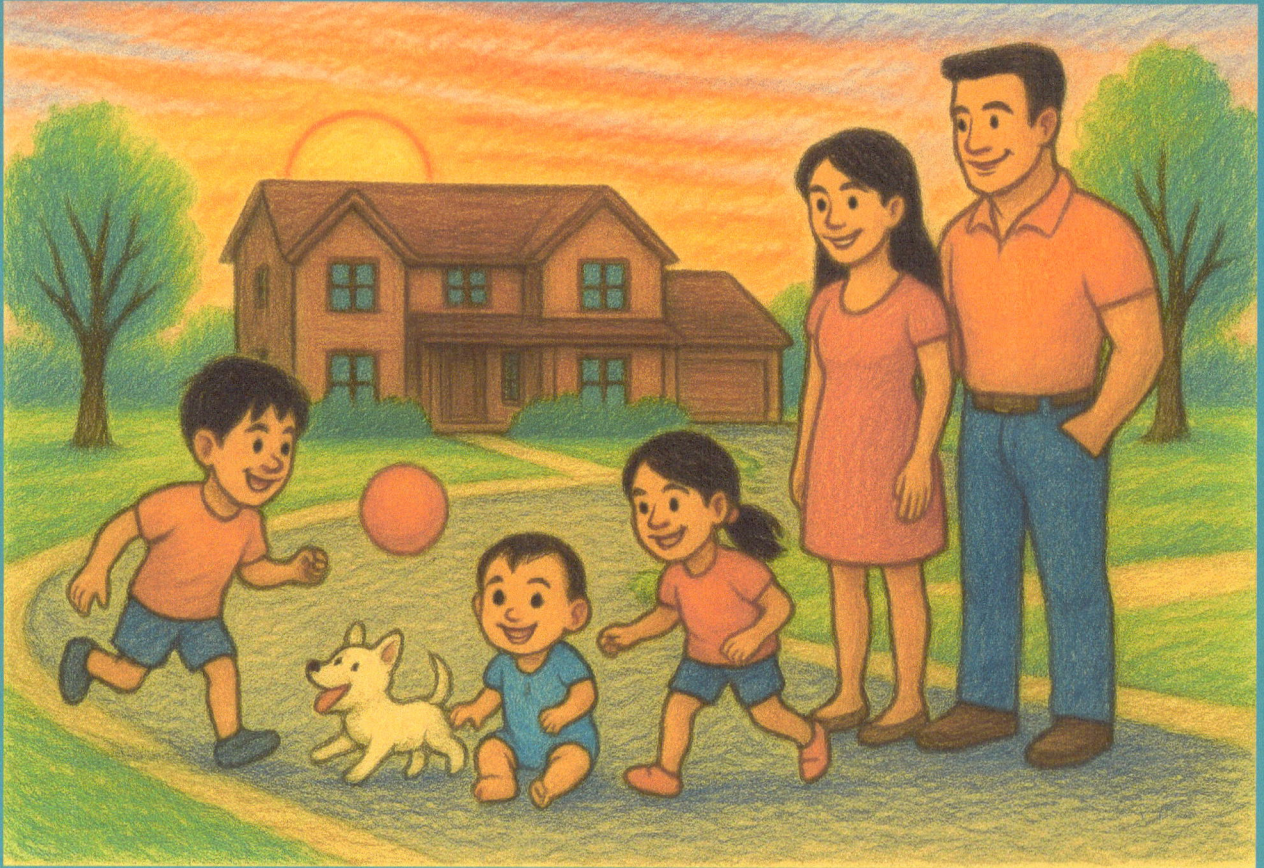

But we are complete with our Special Heart Baby.

AUTHOR'S NOTE

Our third child, Cai, was born in 2024 with Hypoplastic Left Heart Syndrome. It was an unexpected diagnosis that has affected us in both painful and wonderful ways. _____

Cai has had two out of his three open heart surgeries. You can follow his story at heart-glo.org.

We are not sure what the future holds for our family but we know that God is faithful and He has a plan for Cai's life, our special heart baby.

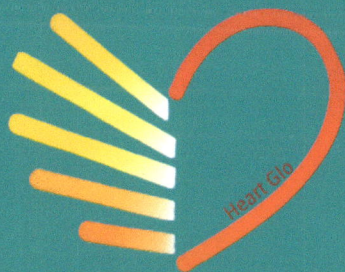

ABOUT THE AUTHOR

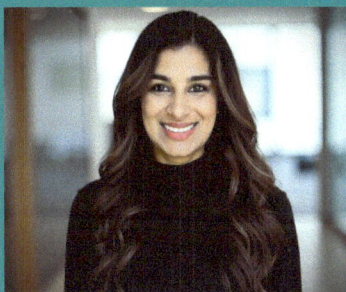

Glory is a wife and mother of three. She has a PhD in cognitive science and an MBA in international management. She works full time in security machine learning and loves to take on new challenges. You can usually find her playing ultimate frisbee with her husband Isaac, riding bikes with Ariella and Benji, or going on walks with Cai.

Glory is nothing without her faith in Jesus. God's love for her and His faithfulness through scripture has given her steadfast hope through all the ups and downs of life. Everything she does and ever wants to be is for His Glory.

Galatians 2:20 "For I have been crucified with Christ, and I no longer live but Christ lives in me. The life I live in the body, I live by faith in the Son of God who loved me and gave Himself for me."

www.ingramcontent.com/pod-product-compliance
Lightning Source LLC
Chambersburg PA
CBHW060818270326
41930CB00002B/83